Dr. Andrew Weil is the leader in the new field of Integrative Medicine, which combines the best ideas and practices of conventional and alternative medicine. A graduate of Harvard Medical School, he is director of the Program in Integrative Medicine at the University of Arizona, the first program to train physicians in this way at an American medical school. He is also the founder of the Center for Integrative Medicine in Tucson, which is advancing the field worldwide. Dr. Weil is well known as an expert in natural medicine, mind-body interactions, and medical botany, as well as the author of the best-selling *Spontaneous Healing* and *8 Weeks to Optimum Health*. According to Dr. Weil, 'Spontaneous healing is not a miracle or a lucky exception, but a fact of biology, the result of the natural healing system that each of us is born with'.

The 'Ask Dr. Weil' program (www.drweil.com) features Andrew Weil, M.D., and is one of the top-rated health sites on the World Wide Web and is featured on Time Warner's Pathfinder Network. The recipient of many awards, it features a daily Q&A with answers to a wide range of health questions, a daily poll, and the Doc Weil Database, which lets readers search hundreds of topics, including material from Dr. Weil's best-selling book *Natural Health, Natural Medicine*. The site also features a Referral Directory (practitioners from acupuncture to Trager work) and DocTalk, a live weekly chat with Dr. Weil. If you have additional questions for Dr. Weil, ask them on his Web site.

By Andrew Weil, M.D.:

Ask Dr. Weil
WOMEN'S HEALTH
YOUR TOP HEALTH CONCERNS
NATURAL REMEDIES
VITAMINS AND MINERALS
COMMON ILLNESSES
HEALTHY LIVING
EATING WELL FOR OPTIMUM HEALTH

8 WEEKS TO OPTIMUM HEALTH
SPONTANEOUS HEALING
NATURAL HEALTH, NATURAL MEDICINE
HEALTH AND HEALING
FROM CHOCOLATE TO MORPHINE
THE MARRIAGE OF THE SUN AND THE MOON
THE NATURAL MIND

Ask Dr. Weil

Vitamins and Minerals

Andrew Weil, M.D.
Edited by Steven Petrow

WARNER BOOKS

All material provided in the *Ask Dr. Weil* program is provided for educational purposes only. Consult your own physician regarding the applicability of any opinions or recommendations with respect to your symptoms or medical condition.

Questions contained in this book may appear in other volumes of the *Ask Dr. Weil* series. The books are arranged according to topic, and to create a complete health profile utilizing Dr. Weil's prescriptions, material may overlap.

A *Warner* Book

First published in Great Britain in 1999 by Warner Books
Reprinted 2000

Published in the United States in 1997 by Ballantine Books, a division of Random House Inc., New York

ISBN 0 7515 2474 3

Typeset in Berkeley by M Rules
Printed and bound in Great Britain by Clays Ltd, St Ives plc

Warner Books
A Division of
Little, Brown and Company (UK)
Brettenham House
Lancaster Place
London WC2E 7EN

Introduction

You've taken the first step toward optimum health. This book will give you more information about my philosophy along with answers to some of the questions I am asked most frequently.

I wrote *Spontaneous Healing* and *8 Weeks to Optimum Health* because I wanted to call attention to the innate, intrinsic nature of the healing process. I've always believed that the body can heal itself if you give it a chance. Why? Because it has a healing system. If you're feeling well, it's important to know about this system so that you can enhance your well-being. If you are ill, you'll also want to know about it because it is your best hope of recovery.

To maintain optimum health requires commitment. This book – and the others in the series – can give you much of the basic information you need about diet, supplements, common illnesses, natural remedies, and healthy living.

All of these questions originated on 'Ask Dr. Weil,' my program on the World Wide Web. If you still have questions, come visit the clinic at www.drweil.com.

What Is Your Antioxidant Cocktail?

Q:
What vitamins should I be taking on a regular basis?

A:
I get asked about the antioxidant 'cocktail' perhaps more than about any other subject. You can really help your body by taking protective antioxidants, nutrients that protect tissues by blocking the chemical reactions by which many toxins cause harm. One way to go about it is to increase your consumption of fresh fruits and vegetables. You can also take supplements.

Here is the formula I use myself and recommend to my patients:

- *Vitamin C:* 1,000 to 2,000 milligrams two to three times a day. Your body can absorb this vitamin more easily in a soluble powder form than in a

1

large tablet. I take a dose of vitamin C with breakfast and dinner, and, if I can remember, another before bed. Plain ascorbic acid may irritate a sensitive stomach, so take it with food or look for a buffered or nonacidic form.

- *Vitamin E:* 400 to 800 IU a day. People under forty should take 400 IU a day; people over forty, 800 IU. Since vitamin E is fat soluble, it must be taken with food to be absorbed. Also, natural vitamin E (d-alpha-tocopherol) is much better than the synthetic form (dl-alpha-tocopherol). I usually take vitamin E at lunch. Make sure the product contains the other tocopherols, especially gamma, which offers protection that alpha-tocopherol does not.

- *Selenium:* 200 to 300 micrograms a day. Selenium is a trace mineral with antioxidant and anticancer properties. Selenium and vitamin E facilitate each other's absorption, so take them together. Vitamin C may interfere with the absorption of some forms of selenium, so take them separately. Doses above 400 micrograms a day may not be healthy.

- *Mixed carotenes:* 25,000 IU a day. I take mixed carotenes as a supplement with my breakfast. I recommend a natural form – easily found in health food stores. Men: read the label to make sure the mixture includes lycopene, the red pigment in tomatoes that helps prevent prostate cancer.

All in all, this is a simple formula that will not cost you too much trouble or money.

3

Do B-12 Boosters Work?

Q:
What do you think of taking B-12 to boost energy? Some friends of mine get shots regularly and say the vitamin works wonders.

A:
B-12 works in the body by helping the bone marrow regenerate red blood cells. The vitamin has been linked to protection against heart disease, and against mental deterioration such as memory loss. People use it to boost their energy, to recuperate from frequent partying with alcohol, and to revitalize themselves during menstruation.

Many people take vitamin B-12 shots as a quick way to pump up their energy level (these are only available on prescription in the U.K.). I see this particularly among entertainers and theater people before performances. But most of them aren't

4

deficient in B-12, so the shots are acting as very effective placebos. A placebo is a medicine or drug that doesn't have any direct therapeutic effect, but because of belief in its effectiveness, the patient experiences benefit. Placebo responses can be extremely powerful, and B-12 shots can definitely elicit them.

Most people I know who get B-12 shots say the first one filled them with a warm glow and a flush of energy. They felt terrific. But subsequent injections don't usually measure up. That's typical of placebos. Extreme fatigue can be a symptom of B-12 deficiency, but that needs to be confirmed by blood tests.

People take B-12 in the form of shots because it's not always easily absorbed through the stomach, and it needs to be combined with calcium to be useful to the body. So injections are the most effective way to get it into your system. If you hate shots, you can take the vitamin as a nasal spray, a nasal gel, or a lozenge you put under your tongue. You can also get it in a time-release formula combined with sorbitol for better absorption through the small intestine.

It's not hard to get enough B-12 in an ordinary diet. The body gets this vitamin almost exclusively from animal sources, such as liver, pork, milk, and eggs. Vegetarians, particularly vegans, are at risk for deficiency, especially vegan children. Many older people have trouble absorbing the vitamin from foods. B-12 deficiency results in pernicious anemia, which can produce such symptoms as weakness, apathy, lightheadedness, shortness of breath, numbness in the extremities, and loss of balance. There may also be accompanying psychiatric changes such as paranoia and depression. In the elderly, B-12 deficiency can cause memory loss and disorientation that may look like Alzheimer's disease. All these symptoms can usually be reversed with supplemental B-12.

Experiment as you wish. B-12 is effective in very small doses, but has been found to be harmless even in amounts much higher than the 6 micrograms recommended daily.

Betting or Bailing on Beta-Carotene?

Q:
I've started to take 20,000 IU of beta-carotene a day per your suggestion. Recently I have read that beta-carotene supplements, even in these modest quantities, can be toxic. What is your latest opinion on the subject?

A:
Beta-carotene is not toxic, and there are no studies that suggest it may be. We do have some new information on the supplement, however, that shows it's not the panacea some people had hoped.

The interest in beta-carotene went mainstream after about two dozen studies showed that people with lots of beta-carotene-rich fruits and vegetables in their diets got less cancer and heart disease. As one of the vitamins that neutralize 'free radical' molecules in the body, beta-carotene seemed to make sense as a preventive to oxidative damage leading to cancer.

7

But the results of giving the vitamin as a supplement were not all encouraging. A Finnish study reported 18 per cent more cases of lung cancer among heavy smokers who took beta-carotene supplements. Then National Cancer Institute researchers halted a study on the effects of beta-carotene and vitamin A. Smokers taking the supplements had 28 per cent more instances of lung cancer than those taking the placebo.

And a twelve-year study of 22,000 physicians found no evidence that beta-carotene supplements were protective against cancer and heart disease.

It's important to note that none of these studies showed that beta-carotene caused cancer. They weren't designed to ask that question. But they do indicate that beta-carotene fails to prevent cancer among smokers. No one is certain why. Some researchers point out that antioxidants can promote free radicals under certain circumstances rather than keeping them under control – and perhaps smoking triggers this action.

It's likely that cancer was already established in the people who were diagnosed with it during these trials. No one believes that antioxidants can cure existing cancers. But study after study has shown the protective effect of high levels of beta-carotene in the blood – and of large amounts of fruits and vegetables in the diet. It is probably not beta-carotene alone that is responsible. It could be the whole family of carotenoid pigments. (And so far, we don't have findings on the effects of beta-carotene in women. The Women's Antioxidant and Cardiovascular Study is continuing despite the negative findings in men.)

We know of about five hundred carotenoids, the family of substances that the body converts into vitamin A. I recommend taking advantage of them all. Eat a diet rich in fruits and vegetables, especially peaches, melons, mangoes, sweet potatoes, squash, pumpkins, tomatoes, and dark leafy greens. And if you cannot include enough of these in your diet, you may want to take a supplement. I recommend a mixed carotene supplement, such as Rainbow Light's Food 4 Life or Schiff's Beta Complete, which contain lycopene, lutein, alpha-carotene, and zeaxanthin, as well as beta-carotene. Take one capsule a day. Men: read labels to be sure the products contain lycopene, the red pigment in tomatoes; recent research shows it can help prevent prostate cancer.

Does Blue-Green Algae Boost Energy?

Q:
I'm curious about the blue-green algae thing. I was a total disbeliever in the high energy and healing claims many people reported to me, but I was worn down by friends and started taking it. It worked! What do you know and think about this?

A:
Frankly, I don't have any firsthand experience with blue-green algae. Like you, I've heard testimonials from people about its energy-boosting effects. According to what I've read, there is very little research on the chemistry or pharmacology of blue-green algae, but I found one unsettling paper indicating that the species used for commercial purposes is capable of producing liver and nerve toxins, which could be unhealthy in long-term use. Many users report drug-like stimulation from these products. Until I know

what's responsible for that effect, I'm not going to recommend them. I've seen dozens of sites on the Web and many print advertisements promoting blue-green algae as a wonder food and an incredible business opportunity. Caveat emptor. I'd say wait and see on this. If it works for you, use it, but keep your eye out for new information.

If low energy is a problem for you, you could consider using ginseng, a natural tonic. Used on a regular basis, ginseng increases energy, vitality, sexual vigor, and provides resistance to all kinds of stress. It is nontoxic but Asian ginseng (*Panax ginseng*) can raise blood pressure and is more of a stimulant. I often recommend American ginseng (*Panax quinquefolius*) to people who are chronically ill and to those lacking in vitality.

How Safe Is Vitamin C?

Q:
Several months ago, the results of carefully planned and carried-out research on human subjects at the National Institutes of Health (NIH) suggested that the RDA for vitamin C should be increased to 200 milligrams a day. Daily intake of more than 800 or 1,000 milligrams may actually be harmful, according to the study. Why have you chosen to stick with your recommendation of 1,000 to 2,000 milligrams a day in the face of these findings?

A:
The doses I suggest are actually very modest doses compared to those recommended by the ultimate vitamin C enthusiast, the late Linus Pauling. He took 18,000 milligrams of vitamin C a day.

I wouldn't go quite that far, but I do recommend 1,000 milligrams twice a day at minimum. We get vitamin C from fruits and vegetables, and we need more of it when exposed to toxins, infection, and chronic illness. If you eat an unhealthy diet or have increased cancer risks for any reason, I'd go up to 2,000 milligrams three times a day. The best form to take is a soluble powder, purchased in bulk (¼ teaspoon equals 1,000 milligrams). I recommend a nonacidic form, because it's easier on your teeth and stomach. Avoid chewable tablets packed with sugar.

I've never seen any toxicity from vitamin C. The only problem that large doses commonly cause is bowel intolerance: flatulence and diarrhea. If this happens, you should just cut back to a more comfortable dose. You can also trigger a deficiency by taking large doses and then stopping suddenly, because the body gets lazy about absorbing it.

The NIH studied absorption of vitamin C into the blood, not its effects on immune function or its ability to counteract degenerative disease. The problem the researchers encountered in doses of about 1,000 milligrams had to do with high production of oxalate, which can spur kidney stones in some people. A magnesium supplement a day can help deter kidney stones, as does remembering to drink plenty of water.

There is one other caution. Recently, doctors have learned that rare individuals suffer from iron overload, usually the result of taking iron supplements or of liver disease. Vitamin C increases the absorption of iron, and high doses can cause serious problems for these individuals.

Some of the advantages of vitamin C, such as the strengthening of blood vessels and connective tissue, do not occur at the levels recommended by the NIH. High vitamin C intake has been linked to denser bones, lowered risk of heart attack, and alleviation of asthma. I don't view vitamin C as a cure for all illnesses, but I do believe we have yet to discover all of its benefits.

The U.S. government approaches setting recommended daily allowances from the perspective of preventing deficiency diseases like scurvy, so the numbers are going to be on the low end. I'm looking at vitamins quite differently – as natural therapeutic agents with a variety of beneficial effects – which is why I consistently recommend more than the RDAs.

Does Vitamin C Aid Recovery from Surgery?

Q:
Have you heard about the intravenous use of vitamin C both before and after surgery to promote faster healing?

A:
Yes. I usually recommend taking 20 grams of vitamin C a day mixed with intravenous fluids, beginning with the IV drip in the operating room and continuing for five days, or until the drip is removed. The problem? Many patients have their requests turned down, either by their doctor or by the hospital pharmacy staff, who are likely to say it's not part of their protocol. Persist. Have your family and friends persist. Say you'll go to another hospital. Then you should be able to get it done. Recently, a friend's brother had surgery for esophageal cancer, and his physician – one of the top gastric surgeons in New York – at first resisted his request for vitamin C, but

15

eventually complied. The result was not surprising to me; the surgeon was so impressed with the speed of healing that he now plans to use vitamin C therapy with other patients.

16

B-6 for Carpal Tunnel Syndrome?

Q:
Due to repetitive typing I have developed carpal tunnel syndrome in both arms. I was given anti-inflammatory medication for this. Then I developed stomach problems – gastritis and irritable bowel syndrome. After two years of getting all kinds of tests done and having doctors tell me that I was going to have to live with this the rest of my life, I got fed up. What do you recommend? Any specific vitamins?

A:
When you're an especially speedy typist or spend long hours at the keyboard, the tendons that move the fingers can swell. There's one little tunnel of ligamentous tissue at the base of your palm that all the tendons and one very important nerve pass through from your arm to your hand. That's where the swelling and pressure can become especially painful

17

and irritating, causing a condition known as carpal tunnel syndrome (CTS).

The most effective treatment that I've found is vitamin B-6 (pyridoxine), 100 milligrams, two or three times a day. In this dosage, pyridoxine is not acting as a B vitamin but rather as a natural therapeutic agent that relieves nerve compression injuries. Be aware that doses of B-6 higher than 300 milligrams a day have caused rare cases of nerve damage. Discontinue usage if you develop any unusual numbness. (A much-publicized University of Michigan study warned about nerve toxicity with B-6 and discouraged people from using it for CTS. I disagree.)

For quick relief when you're hurting, rub on arnica gel, which you can find in your health food store or drugstore. Also, try wrapping ice packs around your wrists (a bag of frozen peas works just as well); if you use this treatment for five minutes every few hours when you're especially stressing your wrists, it may ease the pain and the inflammation. Ginger tablets with DGL (deglycyrrhizinated licorice) may relieve inflammation, and acupuncture certainly can provide symptomatic relief.

The most important consideration when you've got CTS is to figure out ways to reduce your typing. Unless you reduce the strain on your wrists, long-term improvement is unlikely. That means less typing, and learning how to stop driving yourself so hard at the keyboard. There are a couple of other things you can try. Make yourself stand up every hour for a few minutes and stretch. The muscles in your wrists are connected all the way up through your arms, across your shoulders, and up into your neck. Pay attention to those parts of your body, too, because stretching and relaxing your shoulders, neck, and back can ease the strain on your wrists. I know some people who've found a lot of relief through deep-tissue massage or Rolfing. And consider whether you're feeling some emotional tension at work that tightens your whole body, making it more susceptible to injury.

Your posture at the keyboard can make a big difference. Sit up straight, with your weight slightly forward. Your feet should be flat on the floor, or tilted comfortably on an adjustable footrest. An adjustable keyboard tray allows you to change the position of your hands now and then, and helps you keep your wrists straight, with your forearms horizontal and at a 90 degree angle to your upper arms. Your elbows should be at your sides in a relaxed position. Every now and then, tilt your head slowly to each side, and roll your shoulders twice forward and twice back. Squeeze your hands into tight fists and then stretch your fingers out as wide as they will go. Close your hands into fists again and rotate your wrists a few times in either direction.

You may also want to try a different keyboard. Each brand has its own key touches and key widths, some of which may feel better to you than others. If you can find a split keyboard, it may help you keep your hands and arms at a more natural angle. There are also some new keyboards with concave keys, sections tilted up like an accordion, and other unusual shapes. I haven't tried them, but you may want to check them out.

Should Chemo and Antioxidants Be Mixed?

Q:

In your book Spontaneous Healing *you advise discontinuing antioxidants during chemotherapy. My sister, who was diagnosed with ovarian cancer, is scheduled for eight chemo treatments three weeks apart over a twenty-four-week period. Should she discontinue antioxidants for the entire twenty-four weeks, or can she take them after each individual treatment? If so, how soon after each treatment can she start, and how soon before each treatment should she stop?*

A:

You're right. I wrote in *Spontaneous Healing* that 'if you decide to proceed with radiation or chemotherapy, [you should] discontinue use of antioxidant supplements during treatment, since they may protect cancer cells along with normal cells'. In general, antioxidants protect cells from damage by free

21

radicals and other toxins. The safest antioxidants are vitamin C, vitamin E, selenium, and beta-carotene. Together, they block the chemical reactions that create free radicals, which can damage DNA and promote a variety of degenerative changes in cells. Chemotherapy and radiation generate free radicals; that is how they kill dividing cells. By taking antioxidants during chemotherapy, your sister would be reducing the effectiveness of the chemo treatment.

I would discontinue the antioxidants a few days before the start of chemotherapy and stay off them during the entire course of therapy. Then I think your sister could resume within two weeks of chemotherapy. The same holds true with regard to radiation.

Once your sister is finished with chemotherapy, the antioxidants could be helpful. In fact, some studies indicate that antioxidants may help slow the growth of cancerous cells. In addition, cancer is a systemic disease that should be approached from a whole-body perspective. Making a variety of changes to improve one's general health can be very important. Working to heal relationships, keeping up regular exercise, using tonic herbs with immune-enhancing effects, practicing visualization, and taking antioxidants can all help create an environment conducive to optimum health and healing.

By the way, your sister could take immune-protective herbs, such as astragalus, or extracts of reishi or maitake mushrooms during her treatment; they will not interfere with chemotherapy or radiation.

Chromium: Supplement of the Month?

Q:

I've been hearing a lot of talk lately about chromium, both on the news and from some friends in the health business. What exactly does it do, and do you feel it is a beneficial addition to a vitamin diet? Thanks!

A:

You're right, there's a lot of buzz about chromium these days, notably a recent report that chromium produces 'spectacular' results in normalizing glucose and insulin levels in adult-onset diabetes. The U.S. Department of Agriculture study recommended that diabetics take 1,000 micrograms a day.

There's also been a lot of promotion from the manufacturers of one form, chromium picolinate. I often see ads for this product that make unsubstantiated claims like this one:

DIET BOOSTER TABLETS
With Chromium Picolinate

3 STEP FAT ATTACK ...
Appetite Suppressant to
reduce cravings for food.

Fat Metabolizer for efficient metabolic
breakdown of fats, carbs, and proteins.

Diuretic Action assists in
reducing excess fluids.

CHROMIUM PICOLINATE (200 micrograms)
A natural fat metabolizer. This form of
Chromium plays a vital role in the
functioning of insulin responsible for
regulating the efficient metabolism of fats,
carbohydrates, and protein.

These are megaclaims: that chromium will help you lose weight, stabilize blood sugar, treat hypoglycemia, lower cholesterol, and improve blood fats. Unless you're diabetic or deficient in chromium – and most people aren't deficient – I don't think supplemental chromium will do anything for you. This is another example of the supplement-of-the-month mentality that we're seeing all the time. We all want to take a pill to solve our problems, and the manufacturers are ready to sell it to us. Enough said.

What Do You Do with Coenzyme Q?

Q:
What is coenzyme Q and why do you take it?

A:
Coenzyme Q, also known as ubiquinone, is a natural substance found in most foods; it assists in oxygen utilization and energy production by cells, especially heart-muscle cells. Many medical papers demonstrate coenzyme Q's usefulness as a preventive as well as a treatment. In general, coenzymes work with enzymes to help them in their various biochemical functions. Coenzymes are smaller than proteins and so can survive digestion and pass into the system. Coenzyme Q was approved in Japan in 1974 to treat congestive heart failure and has also been approved in Sweden, Italy, Denmark, and Canada. Some people say coenzyme Q increases aerobic endurance, but more studies are needed to verify this. I often recommend it

27

to help stabilize blood sugar in people who have diabetes and to strengthen the heart muscle. It also maintains the health of gums and other tissues. There is evidence that coenzyme Q can prolong survival in women with breast cancer, too.

Your body makes coenzyme Q, and you take it in when you eat fish, meats, and oils from soybean, sesame, and rapeseed. The supplement form is imported from Japan. I take 100 milligrams once a day with food as a general health-booster. Coenzyme Q is harmless, but it's not cheap.

Natural Remedies to Fight a Cold?

Q:
I've spent too much money on all those fancy over-the-counter products for colds. Sometimes they mask the symptoms, but they don't really seem to make me better. Any other recommendations?

A:
You're absolutely right. Most of the over-the-counter products don't help you heal, even if they do stop the sniffles and headaches for a short while. I learned recently that more over-the-counter products are sold for the common cold than for any other disease. Not really surprising. Over the years, I have been collecting home remedies for colds – using myself and my family as guinea pigs. Here's what I've found works best:

Take vitamin C to prevent colds – 1,000 to 2,000 milligrams, three times a day. Start this now if you get more than two colds a year (and add in the rest of my antioxidant cocktail. See page 1).

As soon as you start feeling cold symptoms, eat two cloves (not heads) of raw garlic. Trust me on this. You may not be kissing anyone too soon, but garlic has powerful antibiotic effects. Chop it up and mix it with food, or swallow larger pieces like pills.

You can also take echinacea (*Echinacea purpurea* and related species) at the first sign of a cold or flu – like a scratchy throat or achy back. Take a dropperful of the tincture in a little warm water (or tea) four times a day. Use half doses for children.

Try sucking on zinc gluconate or zinc acetate lozenges, which, according to a recent study, may cut the duration of a cold in half (although zinc acetate may be difficult to find in the U.K.).

Finally, drink this powerful gingerroot tea for head and chest congestion, malaise, and the chills. Here's my recipe:

Grate a 1-inch piece of peeled gingerroot. Put it in a pot with 2 cups of cold water, bring to a boil, lower heat, and simmer five minutes. Add ½ teaspoon cayenne pepper (or more or less to taste) and simmer one minute more. Remove from heat. Add 2 tablespoons of fresh lemon juice, honey to taste, and 1 or 2 cloves of mashed garlic. Let cool slightly, and strain if you desire.

Then get under the covers and drink as much of it as you like. Hope you feel better.

Charmed by Colloidal Minerals?

Q:
How do you feel about taking colloidal mineral supplements?

A:
To me these supplements exemplify obnoxious, multi-level marketing in the name of natural medicine. I've received countless copies of an audiotape that advertises colloidal minerals and makes all sorts of unsubstantiated claims. The veterinarian who pitches the stuff is said to have been nominated for the Nobel Prize in medicine. Well, anyone can write a letter to the Nobel Prize committee. I could nominate you for the Nobel Prize in medicine. I have not seen convincing evidence of therapeutic benefit from taking colloidal minerals. And these products may deliver some substances you definitely don't need – aluminum, for example.

Well, I feel better after venting.

'Colloidal' means the mineral particles are of a certain size, facilitating use by the body. The marketers will tell you that their products make you live twice as long, protect you from cancer, and cure just about anything. They'll tell you that mineral deficiencies lead to a weakened immune system and cancer. You can buy the products as liquid supplements, aerosols, injectables, and vaginal douches. The literature in health food stores says they're powerful antimicrobials and immune-system stimulants; they're supposed to help cure as many as 650 different diseases. None of these claims are proven.

Some colloidal minerals have a long history as medicinals. In the nineteenth century, for example, colloidal silver was promoted as a treatment for everything from colds to rheumatism. Silver products are useful as germicides, but over time they've been replaced by safer and more effective ones.

There is some potential for harm as well. The body doesn't need silver, and the mineral can accumulate in tissues, causing an irreversible bluish discoloration of the skin. There are even some reports of neurological problems in people who have used oral silver products long-term.

Bottom line: I don't recommend colloidal minerals; there's no reason to think they're as good for you as they are for their marketers. Besides, you should be getting your minerals in highly usable form from fruits and vegetables in your diet. Please eat more fruits and vegetables – organically grown, when possible.

Fight Depression Without Drugs?

Q:
What alternatives are there to conventional antidepressant medications or ECT (electroconvulsive or electroshock therapy)? I have tried every medical therapy possible except ECT — but still face recurrent spontaneous episodes of major depression. Are there any alternative treatments that might halt this escalating cycle?

A:
There are only two alternative treatments for depression that I have any confidence in. The first is regular aerobic exercise, which can definitely provide a long-term solution. You'll have to do at least thirty minutes of some vigorous aerobic activity at least five times a week, and be prepared to wait several weeks before you see any benefit. Aerobic exercise is a preventive as well as a treatment.

The second is an herbal treatment, called Saint-John's-wort (*Hypericum perforatum*). Saint-John's-wort is much used in Germany for the treatment of mild to moderate depression, as well as associated disturbed sleep cycles. Take 300 milligrams, three times a day, of a standardized extract containing at least 0.125 per cent hypericin. Again, be prepared to wait two months before you see the full benefit.

Changes in your diet may also make a difference. Try eating less protein and fat, and more starches, fruits, and vegetables. Experiment with the following amino acid and vitamin formula, for which you can find all the ingredients in a health food store. First thing in the morning, take 1,500 milligrams of DL-phenylalanine (DLPA, an amino acid), 100 milligrams of vitamin B-6, and 500 milligrams of vitamin C, along with a piece of fruit or a small glass of juice. Don't eat again for at least an hour. (DLPA can worsen high blood pressure, so use the formula cautiously if you have this condition, and start with a dose of 100 milligrams while monitoring your blood pressure.) Take another 100 milligrams of B-6 and more vitamin C in the evening.

You say you've taken a variety of drugs for depression. In general, I think that the new generation of antidepressants, including Prozac, and U.S. brands Zoloft and Paxil, are less toxic and more effective than medications of the past. Collectively known as SSRIs, or selective serotonin-reuptake inhibitors, they interact with the regulating mechanism for the neurotransmitter serotonin in your brain. It's best to be cautious with any of these drugs, particularly because their makers would have you believe that no one can live a normal life without them.

Make sure you aren't taking any other medications that may contribute to depression. These include antihistamines, tranquilizers, sleeping pills, and narcotics. Recreational drugs, alcohol, and coffee can also make depression worse.

You make reference to ECT – electroconvulsive or electroshock therapy. That is a last resort for the treatment of severe depression. It does work, but I hope things won't get to the point where that's your only option.

Psychiatrists tend to look at all mental problems as stemming from disordered brain chemistry, hence their emphasis on drugs. I believe that disordered moods could just as easily lead to biochemical changes in the brain, so I look elsewhere for treatments. Buddhist psychology views depression as the necessary consequence of seeking stimulation. It counsels us to cultivate emotional balance in life, rather than always seeking highs and then regretting the lows that follow. The prescription is daily meditation, and I agree this may be the best way to get at the root of depression and change it.

Does DHEA Improve Memory?

Q:
My father-in-law takes DHEA along with a few other drugs, all under a doctor's care. He was having trouble remembering things and even being able to carry on a conversation. He says DHEA helps a lot although he doesn't think it is enhancing his memory. What does DHEA do, exactly?

A:
DHEA is a natural hormone produced by the adrenal glands, in the family of male sex hormones. Currently there is great medical interest in the U.S.A. in DHEA (dehydroepiandrosterone), as well as a push from the supplement industry to promote it as an antiaging, antiobesity, anticancer remedy (it is unavailable in the U.K.). Smart-drug enthusiasts think it can also protect brain cells from the degenerative changes of old age. A lot of claims, but not a lot of conclusive science yet.

38

What we do know is that DHEA has a significant anabolic effect, which results in stronger bones and muscles and decreased body fat. It may protect health in a variety of ways. I've seen good results with DHEA in patients with autoimmune diseases like lupus. I also think it might help people with other diseases, such as asthma and rheumatoid arthritis, who have become dependent on prednisone, since it may allow them to wean their bodies off that more dangerous hormone. DHEA is sold as a prescription drug and by several mail-order pharmacies. Health food stores sell DHEA precursors, but those may be worthless. The extracts from wild yams will have no effect, either.

People who tout DHEA point out that we produce most of this hormone in our twenties, with production tapering off in our later years until we produce only about one-fifth as much. They suggest that supplemental DHEA beginning at age forty or fifty could improve quality of life. But evidence for DHEA's benefits is inconclusive. There was one small, six-month study at the University of California–San Diego that reported improved energy and feelings of well-being.

I'm cautious about using any hormones on a regular basis without good reason and without medical supervision. We don't know what the downside of taking supplemental DHEA may be over time. Ray Sahelian, M.D., author of *DHEA: A Practical Guide*, warns against taking high doses cavalierly and suggests consulting with a physician before trying DHEA, because it is a steroid that the body converts into potent estrogens and androgens. Side effects can include acne, facial hair growth in women, deepening of the voice, and mood changes. DHEA probably increases risk of prostate cancer and may increase risk of coronary heart disease.

If your father-in-law's chief concern is his memory, I would suggest an herbal preparation made from the leaves of the ginkgo tree (*Ginkgo biloba*). Researchers have recently begun to study the ability of ginkgo extracts to increase blood flow to the brain. You can buy this nontoxic product in any health food store. Your father-in-law could try taking two tablets or capsules three times a day with meals for memory enhancement. He might not notice any beneficial effects until he has used ginkgo for six to eight weeks.

Getting Enough Folic Acid?

Q:
How important is folic acid? Can't I get this and other B vitamins in a balanced diet?

A:
Folic acid, the synthetic form of the B vitamin folate, is incredibly important. For one thing, folate is a key regulator of an amino acid called homocysteine, a breakdown product of animal protein. A number of studies have connected high levels of homocysteine in the blood to arterial disease and heart attacks. Folate helps the body eliminate homocysteine from the blood. Recently, Dr. Howard Morrison, an epidemiologist in Ottawa, was able to make a direct connection between folate and heart disease. He looked at folate levels in the blood of 5,056 men who had participated in a nutrition study in the 1970s, and he found that those with low levels of the vitamin

were 69 per cent more likely to have died from heart problems in the years since.

Folate also has been found to prevent neural tube defects (such as spina bifida and anencephaly) in babies, which are caused when this structure fails to form properly. The neural tube is the embryonic tissue that later becomes the brain and spinal cord. Apparently folic acid is essential to its proper development. The Food and Drug Administration in the U.S.A. has ordered pasta, rice, and flour makers to add folic acid to their foods by January 1998 as protection against birth defects. This is partly because folic acid plays its important role in neural tube development during the first twenty-eight days of conception – usually before the woman knows she is pregnant – so it doesn't help to tell women to take vitamin supplements during pregnancy.

Folate also may be involved in preventing a whole range of chronic diseases. As the folic acid fortification rule moves into place, we may see a number of health benefits. In fact, since the Morrison study, some doctors are saying the government should double its folic acid RDA (recommended daily allowance), from 200 micrograms to 400 micrograms, to help people protect their hearts.

Folic acid is abundant in dark-green leafy vegetables, carrots, torula yeast, orange juice, asparagus, beans, and wheat germ. But as many as 90 per cent of

Americans don't get that protective 400 micrograms in their diet – for example, you'd have to eat two cups of steamed spinach, a cup of boiled lentils, or eight oranges every day. So it's important to take a supplement, especially if you're a woman and considering having children someday.

A few cautions, though: Some people are allergic to the folic acid in pills. Also, anyone with a history of convulsive disorder or hormone-related cancer should not take doses above 400 micrograms a day for extended periods. Finally, high levels of folate can mask the signs of vitamin B-12 deficiency. Older people and vegetarians, who are most at risk for deficiencies in B-12, should make sure they're also getting enough of that vitamin if they begin taking folic acid supplements.

Ginger as an Anti-Inflammatory?

Q:
You recommended ginger to cure wrist tendinitis. I have some tendinitis in both of my wrists and also am beginning to have pains in my lower thumb joints. I have been consuming large amounts of cooked ginger in a fried form. Is this the amount that should make a detectable difference? (I am talking about thin slices of a knob or two of a piece of ginger.)

A:
You may not be getting enough of ginger's anti-inflammatory effect with the cooked fresh ginger. The preferred form for this use is the powder. My preference would be to start with one capsule of 500 milligrams of ginger twice a day with food. You can go up to two capsules twice a day with food. You can also use as much fresh ginger as you like in preparing your food. But keep in mind that fresh ginger is not as

44

rich in anti-inflammatory components as dried ginger.

Ginger's effect on inflammation is documented in several studies. A possible mechanism of action involves a change in the synthesis of prostaglandins and leucotrienes – hormones that mediate inflammation.

Ginger is usually called a root, but it's actually a rhizome, an underground stem of a tropical plant, *Zingiber officinale*. Besides having anti-inflammatory properties, ginger works well as a treatment for nausea and motion sickness – probably the use for which it is most valued. Its efficiency is attributed to the volatile oil that gives ginger its characteristic pungency. Ginger also tones the cardiovascular system and reduces platelet aggregation, helping to protect against heart attacks and strokes.

Why the Wait for Herbal Benefits?

Q:
In many of your discussions about vitamins and herbs you say it may take up to two months before you see results. Why does it take so long before we can notice any benefits?

A:
As a society we're used to taking purified drugs, powerful agents that typically produce immediate effects. When you're using herbal treatments, you're working with dilute, much weaker preparations. Natural remedies require you to think about health and medicine in a different way. We've become conditioned by pharmaceuticals to expect quick, dramatic responses in our bodies. But often, these drugs are only suppressing symptoms, rather than treating the root problem. With natural medicine, you're reaching more deeply into the body's systems to create lasting health.

46

Herbs often contain families of active ingredients, instead of one concentrated, powerhouse chemical. They may include elements that soften the impact of the main component, or that create other effects. There are important differences between taking a caffeine tablet and drinking a cup of coffee. Or snorting cocaine instead of chewing on a coca leaf.

Often when you use herbs and vitamins as remedies, you're working to change body chemistry and physiology, rather than simply suppress symptoms. In order to see the more profound changes, a certain amount of time is required. And often the changes will be subtle.

Some herbal treatments and other natural remedies can work quickly. One example is stinging nettle (*Urtica dioica*), for hay fever. It relieves symptoms rapidly and without toxicity, with the added bonus of providing trace minerals. Other speedy solutions include the ancient medicinal plant ephedra (*Ephedra sinica*), for acute asthma attacks, and licorice extract (not red licorice twists!), for stomach distress. And when you get a cold or the flu, you can expect echinacea, the purple coneflower (*Echinacea purpurea*), to help out quickly. But in many cases, such as when using Saint-John's-wort (*Hypericum perforatum*) to treat depression, it can take six to eight weeks before you notice changes. It may also take that long for you to be reasonably sure it's the herb making the difference, not a visit from a friend or a pleasant surprise at work. With any of these herbs, you may see results sooner, but my point is to be patient when you're using natural remedies.

Can I Take an Herbal Overdose?

Q:
I would like to know whether there is any herb that one could consume to excess and therefore suffer health problems. I consume 25 grams of raw ginger, 25 grams of raw garlic, and 20 grams of eleuthero (Siberian ginseng) every day. Are there any dangers in doing so? I also plan to take triphala, ashwagandha, barley green, sun chlorella, echinacea, Ginkgo biloba, and gotu kola. Is there any harm in taking any of these products in the same or larger quantities?

A:
That's a lot of herbs to take every day, and I have to wonder what health problems you're using them for. In general, I think it's a shame to waste medicinal herbs by taking them just because they're there. They'll work better for you if you save them for the times when your body needs special attention.

I think any herb can be taken in excess. For example, there have been a few reported cases of bleeding problems in people taking very large amounts of garlic, which can act as an anticoagulant. Some herbalists also say that too much garlic can deplete your intestinal flora and make it harder to absorb nutrients.

I think the amounts of ginger and garlic you're talking about are fine. But I wonder about swallowing a whole grab bag of herbs, unless you're taking them for specific reasons.

Herbs are dilute forms of natural drugs, not health foods or dietary supplements. You shouldn't take them casually or for no reason, any more than you would take pharmaceutical drugs casually or for no reason. Any herb that produces a therapeutic effect can also cause side effects. And, just as for any drug, it's important to watch for sensitivities particular to your body.

Unless you have specific illnesses you are treating, I'd back off from the herbal cornucopia. If you use herbs just because you think it's healthy to do so, you may build up a resistance to their effects. Then you won't have them available to work for you if you get sick and really need them.

Help for Hot Flushes?

Q:
I have tried herb after herb and I still can't find the right combination to get rid of my hot flushes. I'm desperate. Can you help?

A:
It's interesting how medicine has transformed a natural phase in the cycle of women's bodies into a disorder. For many years, it was considered impolite to even mention the word (that's when menopause was referred to as 'the change'). Then menopause became one in a long list of imbalances attributed to women's reproductive systems, with proper intervention mandated. Pharmaceutical companies and gynecologists bombard women with the same message: Menopause is a time of unhappiness, bringing moodiness, hot flushes, osteoporosis, and loss of youthful attractiveness. The 'life change' is actually a

deficiency disease, the theory goes, and so only estrogen replacement therapy can restore vibrancy to women's bodies.

I'd recommend looking at this time of life in a new way. Instead of signifying aging and the loss of childbearing ability, menopause can be a time to discover new energy, a freer self, and deeper wisdom within. Yes, there are discomforts associated with the changes in your body during this time. But these are signs of an opportunity to discover and claim the power of the second half of life.

During menopause, your body is adjusting to a change in hormone production. The ovaries stop releasing eggs, and it's no longer possible to get pregnant. The pituitary hormones, follicle-stimulating hormone (FSH), and luteinizing hormone (LH), which normally cycle during the month, begin to flow continuously at high levels. The ovaries slow down their output of estrogen, progesterone, and androgens. At the same time, other sites, such as the adrenal gland, the skin, and the brain, may take over hormone production. The ease of the transition depends greatly on a woman's stress level, emotional health, and nutritional status.

We rarely hear about women who have few problems with menopause, even though there are many of them. In non-Western cultures, menopause is often considered a time of strengthening and health for women. So first of all, it's important not to buy into the negative images and attitudes surrounding menopause in our culture.

Around 85 per cent of American women experience the hot flushes you mention during menopause. Not long ago, Jane Fonda described her first hot flush this way: 'When Ted and I were courting at a sound-and-light show in Athens, Greece, I had my first hot flush. It was dramatic and kind of exciting'. You may feel a great heat around your head and neck, sweat profusely, then feel chilled. Some women go through these episodes for a few months, some for years. Hot flushes have been linked to blocked energy and unused sexual potential, so women who fear they will lose their sex drive with menopause may be more bothered by them. One tactic is to work to free your sexual energy and overcome the messages you are getting about an expected loss of sex drive.

I personally recommend a menopausal formula that works well for most women. Buy capsules or tinctures of these herbs at a health food store: dong quai, a female tonic made from the root of *Angelica sinensis*; vitex, or chaste tree (*Vitex agnus-castus*), a regulator of the female reproductive system; and damiana (*Turnera diffusa*), a plant that has a reputation as a tonic and female aphrodisiac. Take two capsules of each of these every day at noon, or one dropperful of each tincture mixed in warm water once a day at noon. Keep taking the herbs until you don't experience any hot flushes, then begin to reduce the dose and try to stop altogether.

Another herb widely used for menopausal discomforts, including hot flushes, is black cohosh (*Cimifuga racemosa*), now available in the U.S.A. as a commercial product called Remifemin. Its effectiveness is supported by good scientific data.

Many women also find ginseng to be very helpful for hot flushes, especially in combination with vitamin E (800 IU a day of the natural form). Nutrition is also important. Soy products contain estrogenlike substances that may account for the low incidence of menopausal symptoms in Japanese women. And researchers have found that deep, slow breathing can reduce hot flushes by half, probably by calming the central nervous system.

Finally, there are other Chinese herbs that help to relieve the problem. I'd suggest you visit a practitioner of traditional Chinese medicine if you want to learn about them.

Do Marijuana Users Need Additional Vitamins?

Q:

What vitamins would you recommend to keep an otherwise healthy marijuana smoker in the best shape? I've heard that marijuana depletes certain vitamins in the body.

A:

If you use any drug (alcohol, amphetamines, barbiturates, cocaine, narcotics, or marijuana), I would recommend taking a B-complex supplement every day in addition to a basic antioxidant formula (see page 1).

This cocktail helps protect your immune and healing systems, giving your body an edge against all kinds of irritation, including that produced by smoking anything – marijuana or tobacco. Medical evidence for the beneficial effects of antioxidant vitamins and minerals keeps accumulating. In addition, drink plenty of water (everyone should drink six to eight glasses a day) and try to breathe fresh air as often as possible.

Latest on Melatonin?

Q:

What do you think of melatonin? Is 3 milligrams a normal dose?

A:

Melatonin is the first and only effective remedy for jet lag, and I recommend it, for that purpose (it's even effective for west-to-east travel, which many people find harder). It's also useful as an occasional remedy for insomnia – especially for people working shifts – or for disturbed sleep cycles. If you go through periods where you're dead tired at 7 P.M. and then find yourself wide awake at, say, 11 P.M., melatonin might change your cycle, allowing you to go to sleep at a better time and sleep for the whole night. For these uses, taking melatonin for only one or two nights might be sufficient.

But evidence for melatonin's effects as an immune-booster and a chemical fountain of youth is lacking –

popular books and articles notwithstanding. Because it is a brain hormone, secreted by the pineal gland, with very general effects on the body, I'm wary about recommending it for use on a regular basis over long periods of time.

You should also know that the quality of melatonin products on the market is uneven, and many dosage forms are too high. A 1-milligram tablet taken sublingually (under the tongue) is probably more than enough for any use. The best book on the topic is *Melatonin*, by Russel J. Reiter, Ph.D., and Jo Robinson.

How Good Are Multivitamins?

Q:
I'd like your opinion on multivitamins. I'm in good health but often can't eat right. Is a good multi advisable? And if so, what should I look for? Is there any difference between different brands of the exact same vitamins? What's the best way to compare them?

A:
If you're not eating regularly, if your diet is not rich in fresh foods, and if you don't get plenty of fruits and vegetables, a multivitamin is an easy solution. It's better to take your vitamin cocktail in stages throughout the day, but I'm not opposed to taking your daily requirement all at once in one capsule, pill, or tablet after your biggest meal.

Some precautions: I would check the doses to make sure you're getting enough antioxidants. That would be 25,000 IU beta-carotene (preferably with

59

other carotenes such as alpha-carotene, lutein, zeaxanthin, and lycopene), 400 IU of natural vitamin E (twice that much if you're over forty), and 2,000 milligrams of vitamin C, plus 200 micrograms of selenium a day. If not, take extra supplements to make up the difference.

It's also possible to get too much of some things in a multivitamin. You don't want more than 400 micrograms a day of folic acid, because then you risk masking a vitamin B-12 deficiency without added benefits from the folic acid. And make sure there's no iron in there if you're not a woman of menstruating age or a person with proven iron-deficiency anemia. Iron is an oxidizing agent that can promote cancer and heart disease, and the body has no way of eliminating excess amounts except through blood loss.

I don't think those vitamin packs are worth it. You can make up your own packs, if you want. Or if it's the convenience you're after, a multivitamin probably makes more sense.

In general, when shopping for the vitamins, there really aren't any buzzwords to look for. Just use the same common sense you might use when looking for a bottle of juice for lunch or the right flour for the bread you're baking. You want products free of dyes, preservatives, and nonessential additives. And you might as well check out the cheapest ones that are free of additives first.

Read the labels. See whether the vitamin is in the form you like – a big capsule, a soft gel capsule, or a tablet. Look at the dose, and make sure the cheapest isn't just a lower amount of the vitamin encased in the same number of tablets. And make sure you know the desired dose. For instance, you can buy a calcium supplement only to find out you need six tablets in order to get the dose you want. Once I got a B-50 B-complex home and then realized that it provided only 200 milligrams a day of folic acid – half the daily amount I recommend.

Generally, the difference between natural and synthetic vitamins is not important. An exception is vitamin E. Most of the vitamin E you see on store shelves is synthetic, noted as dl-alpha-tocopherol on the label. Don't buy it. Instead, go for natural vitamin E, or d-alpha-tocopherol, combined with other tocopherols. Once you find a brand you like for a particular vitamin, stick with it.

You'll find there are enormous differences in pricing. It's worth doing some research to find reliable, low-priced sources.

Seeking News on Selenium?

Q:
I've been reading a lot about selenium in the newspaper these days. Can it really prevent cancer?

A:
The recent study about selenium that came out of the University of Arizona caused quite a stir. For a long time, people have believed that selenium protects against cancer, heart ailments, and other diseases. But studies on the subject were in disagreement. So the Arizona Cancer Center at the University of Arizona in Tucson, where I teach, planned a randomized trial to study the ability of selenium supplements to protect against two skin cancers: basal cell carcinoma and squamous cell carcinoma. Dr. Larry Clark and a team of researchers recruited 1,312 patients from the eastern coastal plain of the United States, where selenium levels in the soil and crops are low, and skin cancer

rates are high. All of the patients had a history of the disease. Half of the group received sugar pills every day for an average of 4.5 years, and the other half took 200 micrograms of selenium in supplement form each day.

Clark found that the selenium supplements didn't have any effect on skin cancers. But halfway through the study, the researchers decided to look at other types of cancers and cancer mortality in general. At the end of the study, they had some dramatic results. The people who had taken selenium had 63 per cent fewer prostate cancers, 58 per cent fewer colorectal cancers, and 46 per cent fewer lung cancers than the rest of the group. Overall, there were 39 per cent fewer new cancers among those taking selenium. And altogether, half as many died from their cancer. The selenium seemed to be so beneficial, the researchers stopped the blinded phase of the trial early.

There are several possible mechanisms for the protective effect of selenium. Selenium activates an enzyme in the body called gluthathione peroxidase that protects against the formation of free radicals – those loose molecular cannons that can damage DNA. In this situation, selenium may work interchangeably (and in synergy) with vitamin E. In test tube studies, selenium inhibited tumor growth and regulated the natural life span of cells, ensuring that they died when they were supposed to instead of turning 'immortal' and hence malignant. Because of this particular action, the University of Arizona researchers say that selenium could be effective within a fairly short time frame.

There were some weaknesses in this study, among them the fact that few women were included. Because the results are not consistent with those of other studies (using lower doses), the researchers and other cancer specialists are calling for further randomized trials before any national recommendations are made about selenium supplementation.

I'm all for that. But in the meantime, I will continue to take my 200 micrograms of selenium a day – the same dose used in the study – and I suggest that you do, too. Excess selenium has been associated with toxicity, so don't go overboard. If you're not fond of popping pills, you can get 120 micrograms of selenium in just one Brazil nut. Buy the shelled kind – they're grown in a central region of Brazil where the soil is richest in the mineral. Other good sources are tuna fish, seafood, wheat germ, and bran.

A Proven Sex-Drive Enhancer?

Q:
Is there anything I can take to boost my sex drive? I'm female.

A:
Of course, people have been asking this question for centuries. Curiously enough, a proven sex-drive enhancer for women is the male hormone testosterone. Women produce their own testosterone, and reputable scientific studies show that tiny additional amounts can increase libido dramatically. One testosterone product, formulated in the U.S.A. for women in menopause, is called Estratest (unavailable in the U.K.); it also contains estrogen.

An herbal possibility for women is the Mexican plant damiana (*Turnera diffusa*), which has a reputation as a female aphrodisiac. Not that much is known about it, but you can find damiana preparations in health food stores. Again, follow dosage recommendations on the label. Whichever of these appeals to you, try it for a few months and see what it can do for you. If it works, great. If not, there's no point in continuing the treatment.

But before spending money on substances like these, you might want to consider other ways to boost sexual energy. Both physical and mental well-being are important to healthy sex. Think about the interplay of emotional charge, mental imagery, and body responses associated with sex. Hypnotherapy and guided imagery therapy can help you make the most of the mind-body connection in overcoming sexual problems. Many experts, myself included, say the greatest aphrodisiac is the human mind.

Cancer-Killing Sharks?

Q:
What do you know about cancer patients using shark cartilage? How does it work to help treat the cancer?

A:
Shark cartilage has become popular as an arthritis treatment and a therapy for cancer and AIDS. I haven't seen any good scientific evidence that it works, just anecdotal reports and suggestive laboratory studies. The theory is that shark cartilage contains substances that inhibit the proliferation of new blood vessels that tumors need in order to continue to grow. Mainstream scientists have isolated several compounds from shark tissue, notably squalamine, that do have this effect. But the shark antitumor substances they are investigating aren't found in the cartilage. Furthermore, even if there are beneficial substances in the cartilage, I'm not

convinced the commercial capsules provide them in a form the body can absorb.

Most scientists object strongly to the intense promotion and commercialization of shark cartilage because there is so little evidence of its efficacy. Meanwhile, its popularity has helped decimate shark populations.

When considering alternative treatments for cancer, it's wise to seek good published data on outcomes from their use. If you can't find published data, ask to see statistical data from providers. Look particularly for any risk of toxicity or harm. And finally, ask to talk with patients who have undergone the alternative therapy. If you have cancer, it is important to work to improve overall health and resistance on all levels. A book on alternative cancer therapies I recommend to my cancer patients is *Choice in Healing*, by Michael Lerner.

Energized by Wheatgrass?

Q:
What do you think of wheatgrass? I've heard that 1 ounce supposedly contains as much nutritional value as 2.5 pounds of vegetables. Is that true?

A:
Wheatgrass is a sprouted grain that grows naturally in pastures. Cattle love it – but only when it's nice and green. These days, you're likely to see gardens of wheatgrass in juice bars and health food stores, along with green powders and tablets. Wheatgrass enthusiasts use juice from the young shoots in all sorts of ways, from juice drinks to enemas. They use it as part of a regimen for treating cancer and for building up the body's immunity.

Wheatgrass is supposed to have high life energy and many other positive attributes. You'll find claims that it will clean your blood, repair your DNA,

69

deodorize your body, keep your hair from turning gray, help your pet, confer energy, and lengthen your life. The chlorophyll is supposed to act as an antioxidant and the nutrients are thought to provide an energy lift.

Unfortunately, despite wheatgrass's wide popularity, there's no evidence to back any of these claims. And I don't recommend its use other than as a source of minerals and vitamins. If you like wheatgrass and it appeals to you, fine. Drink it. But I don't think it's a substitute for 2.5 pounds of vegetables. Besides, I don't like the way it tastes.

Yams for Hormone Therapy?

Q:
What's the scoop on wild yam cream? Is it merely a marketing phenomenon? Or does it have real botanical benefits for PMS sufferers and menopausal discomfort relief-seekers?

A:
Wild yam, or *Dioscorea*, is the tuber of a tropical plant. Don't expect to find it in your grocery store – it's completely unrelated to the sweet potatoes that many people call yams in this country. All sorts of claims have been made about wild yam because it contains a precursor of steroid hormones called diosgenin, which was used as the starting material for the first birth control pill. But diosgenin itself has no hormonal activity. Nor can the human body convert it into something that does.

That's why I question the efficacy of creams that

71

contain only wild yam as the supposed source of natural hormonal activity. Some of these creams may contain a natural form of progesterone synthesized from diosgenin, even though this doesn't show up on the label. That would certainly make them active.

Wild yam may have sedative properties that can help relieve premenstrual problems. In *Herbs for Health and Healing*, Kathi Keville recommends a tea made of 1 teaspoon vitex berries, 1 teaspoon wild yam, ½ teaspoon each of burdock root, dandelion root, feverfew leaves, and the flowering parts of hops. Place the herbs in a pot containing a pint and a half of water and bring to a boil. Then steep for at least twenty minutes with the heat off. It may help with the cramps, emotional changes, and nausea you sometimes feel before your menstrual period. You can also buy a tincture with these herbs.

Can Zinc Cure the Common Cold?

Q:
I've heard some talk about zinc lozenges as a cure for the common cold. Is there any validity to this claim? If it's true where can I find the lozenges?

A:
Zinc gluconate lozenges do have a lot of enthusiasts, although in my experience, reports from users vary. Research on zinc has also delivered mixed results, but one recent study at the Cleveland Clinic found the mineral to cut the duration of a cold in half. No one, however, has found a cure for the common cold.

In the Cleveland study, 50 people with colds sucked on Cold-Eeze lozenges (13 milligrams each) every two hours. Their symptoms cleared up four days sooner than the coughing, runny noses, and sore throats of a comparable group that didn't use the lozenges. Michael Macknin, who designed the research, thinks

73

the zinc ions traveled from the mouth to the nose, where they prevented the viruses that cause colds from settling into the respiratory pathways.

You should be aware that daily doses of zinc above 100 milligrams may depress immunity. And zinc can upset some people's stomachs, so make sure you've eaten before sucking on the lozenges. A lot of people don't like the taste of the lozenges, either.

I personally haven't experienced great benefits from zinc lozenges, but I think they are worth trying. You can buy them in health food stores or regular drugstores. Some say that the newer zinc acetate lozenges work better than standard forms (although these may be difficult to find in the U.K.).

Resources

Books by Andrew Weil, M.D.

8 Weeks to Optimum Health: A Proven Program for Taking Full Advantage of Your Body's Natural Healing Power. London: Little, Brown, 1997.

Spontaneous Healing: How to Discover and Enhance Your Body's Natural Ability to Maintain and Heal Itself. London: Little, Brown, 1995.

Natural Health, Natural Medicine: A Comprehensive Manual for Wellness and Self-Care. Rev. ed. London: Little, Brown, 1997.

Health and Healing: Understanding Conventional and Alternative Medicine. Rev. ed. Boston: Houghton Mifflin, 1995.

From Chocolate to Morphine: Everything You Need to Know About Mind-Altering Drugs, with Winifred Rosen. Rev. ed. Boston: Houghton Mifflin, 1993.

The Natural Mind: An Investigation of Drugs and the Higher Consciousness. Rev. ed. Boston: Houghton Mifflin, 1986.

The Marriage of the Sun and the Moon: A Quest for Unity in Consciousness. Boston: Houghton Mifflin, 1980.

Other Recommended Books

Fulford, Robert C., and Gene Stone. *Dr. Fulford's Touch of Life: The Healing Power of the Natural Life Force*. New York: Pocket Books, 1996.

Keville, Kathi, with Peter Korn. *Herbs for Health and Healing: The Illustrated Encyclopedia of Herbs*. Emmaus, Pennsylvania: Rodale Press, 1996.

Lerner, Michael. *Choice in Healing: Integrating the Best of Conventional and Alternative Approaches to Cancer*. Cambridge: MIT Press, 1994.

Northrup, Christiane, M.D. *Women's Bodies, Women's Wisdom: Creating Physical and Emotional Health and Healing*. New York: Bantam Books, 1995.

Reiter, Russel J., and Jo Robinson. *Melatonin: Your Body's Natural Wonder Drug*. New York: Bantam Books, 1995.

Sahelian, Ray, M.D. *DHEA: A Practical Guide*. Garden City Park, New York: Avery Publishing Group, 1996.

Program in Integrative Medicine

At the University of Arizona Health Sciences Center, Tucson, Arizona. For more information, visit the Web site: http://www.ahsc.arizona.edu/integrative_medicine. Or write: Center for Integrative Medicine, P.O. Box 64089, Tucson, AZ 85718.

Newsletter

If you would like more information on my lectures and informational products, including my monthly newsletter, *Self Healing*, please write to: Andrew Weil, M.D., P.O. Box 457, Vail, AZ 85641.

On the Web

'Ask Dr. Weil' answers health questions daily on Time Warner's Pathfinder Network (www.drweil.com).

Index

Index

Index

Index

Acknowledgments

Richard Pine, Judith Curr, Elisa Wares and Scott Fagan